WORKBOOK

For

THE BODY KEEPS THE SCORE

BRAIN, MIND, AND BODY IN THE HEALING OF TRAUMA

BESSEL VAN DER KOLK, MD

Roger Press

ISBN: 978-1-952663-77-2
Made in Colors Publishers

Table of Contents

INTRODUCTION: FACING TRAUMA

This book attempts to comprehend how humans continue to stay alive and heal completely after each traumatic experience. The author meticulously gathered facts from years of brainstorming and study with colleagues and working alongside men, women, and children that are traumatized to know how the body, mind, and brain functions and heals from traumatic experiences.

Traumatic experiences occur in our everyday life, child abuse, rape, physical violence, and many more. Limiting traumatic events to bomb blast and very gory human-induced large scale homicide is not a way to look at these experiences. Humans have been sturdy over the years and even amid physical and emotional pain. But, these traumatic events leave their traces behind. It sticks like a leech to our emotions, ecology, immune system, and even hinders our ability to be joyful and intimate.

Traumatized people try hard to convince their brain that they can survive what they have experienced but immediately the brain senses any similar danger, the entire system dispatches a quantifiable amount of stress hormone that triggers hostile emotions, strong physical perceptions, and violence. Currently, the functionality of the body system (organ) is easily spelled out by medical practitioners but what hasn't been figured is the complexity of the human mind and what goes on in the brain, and what compels love.

Three scientific studies have generated new disciplines to help us understand the effects of neglect, psychological trauma, and abuse. They are **neuroscience, developmental psychopathology, and interpersonal neurobiology**. The first discipline concerns how our brain backs up mental progressions, the second term developmental psychopathology concerns itself with the level of impact the hostile experience hampers on the brain and mind development, while the last term; interpersonal neurobiology studies the level in which our behavior affects the ecology, mindset, and emotions of our immediate environment.

These disciplines reveal that trauma hugely affects the area of the brain that struggles for survival. It also leads to physical alterations, remodeling the alarm system of the brain, a significant increase in the stress-induced hormone, and changes in the system that sieves significant information from the irrelevant. So, next time you want to breathe down on a traumatized individual for repeatedly practicing the same odd thing; know that it is tied to involuntary changes that occurred in their brain due to the trauma they suffered.

There are ways to alleviate the impact of a traumatic experience. First – talk and reach out; don't die in silence, let those around know what you are going through. Another way is by taking medications that turn off unnecessary alarm feedback or adopt methods that will enable the brain to process information aright. Lastly, another method is to flood the traumatized with experiences opposite from what they have suffered that usually makes them helpless and angry. Each survivor's experience is peculiar to them. They need to lord over their trauma and grab their lives back. This piece provides a comprehensive explanation as to the technique to adopt to recover completely after a traumatic attack.

PART ONE: THE REDISCOVERY OF TRAUMA
CHAPTER 1: LESSONS FROM VIETNAM VETERANS

Bessel van der Kolt's first professional encounter with a Vietnamese veteran was in July 1978 at the Boston Veterans Administration Clinic. There he met Tom, their conversation was filled with horrible and hurtful experiences of what Tom had suffered in his time of service, how he is still reliving it in nightmares and flash memories. This made him aggressive and hostile to his family and he finally withdrew from them. The author who could relate was also born during the postwar times in Holland where he would play in buildings that were blasted. To make matters worse he had a father who was constantly against the Nazis.

Bessel noticed the same trace of intensified anger and disconnection in his dad and uncle, which was also evident in Tom sitting before him. Bessel, a Medical student who studied sleep cycles prescribed a psychoactive drug to help Tom sleep better and horde off his nightmares. To his surprise at their next meeting, Tom didn't use the drug and his excuse was that the drug will make him forget his dead friends and that will make their death for nothing. Bessel was irritated but he noted that the state of the dead still had a huge effect on the living and therefore hindered him from moving forward in life.

Trauma has a lot of mysteries surrounding it that will take a lifetime of discovery to fully comprehend why people stay stuck in the ugly events of the past. What goes on in their brains and minds that keep them trapped for centuries? And why is it hard to let go and take rightful ownership of their lives once again? Looking at Tom who found a way of ending his constant suffering (at least temporarily for a start) refused help in other to keep the memory of his dead compatriots alive and burning inside of him. For a long time, there were no materials on war neurosis, battle fatigue, shell shock, or anything related to what patients with trauma feel exactly and how they can be truly helped. Later in 1941 a publication on *The Traumatic Neuroses of War* by Abram Kardiner explained the presence of similar emotions in war veterans as pointed out by Bessel which were the feeling of vainness and withdrawal. These were the feeling of traumatic neuroses referred to as posttraumatic stress disorder (PTSD) today. Kardiner identified that PTSD makes its victims unnecessarily nervous and hypervigilant to threat, so it is not a mind thing but doused with physical properties. So how can veterans be helped?

Facing reality is hard, but the truth is – it is an excruciating self-torture to lie to yourself for long. Have we intentionally inquired what these trauma survivors go through? Is it a sincere concern to know the truth of what hurts them even though we get to be hurt in between? Or we force ourselves to believe it is rosy and safe for people anywhere when you and I know the truth. It is pertinent and important to help in restoring the days when life was worthwhile back into the traumatized.

TRAUMA AND THE LOSS OF SELF

A traumatic event can be a result of another person's action affecting you or one that is self-inflicted ensuing from a tragic experience. Detailed experience of the traumatized Veterans has a big role to play in finding back themselves. These are people who used to be sweet, loving, great friends, and warm family members. Now they are a shadow of themselves as their experience has numbed the part of their emotions that makes them good, rational, and human.

A traumatized individual cannot be intimate, trust others, or even be trusted after the gruesome things you've done? This experience is in two ways, you feel enraged because you could have fought your ways out of the predicament or that you could have done something differently, but fright couldn't allow you man up to a fellow human like yourself; now you are hunted for eternity with the thought streaming your conscious and subconscious mind now and then.

Shame is also associated with trauma especially when he/she has to keep relating to their abuser. For example, a victim of child abuse whose violator is a close relation.

NUMBING

This is a feeling not farfetched in survivors. Distancing yourself in other not to harm those you love isn't the solution to curb the trauma demons. When Tom realized that through the help of Bessel, Tom went back home to his wife and children.

THE REORGANIZATION OF PERCEPTION

How does trauma alter individual perceptions and thoughts? A typical experience occurred with Bill a medic who had witnessed the war in Vietnam and spent every day relieving all he had seen and heard. An inkblot test was carried out called "Rorschach" which uniquely reveals what is in the mind. In that test, it revealed that Bill was still seeing the faces of dead children that were blown up, blood trailing down the gutter and over the faces of injured survivors.

The horror displayed by Bill only reinforced the longing to find solutions to the agony faced by these traumatized folks. Hurtful memories don't take permission before creeping in and you cannot stop them from playing in your mind's eye. Our perception has a crucial role to play on how we interpret things. It is observed that people with trauma play a good role in overlaying their trauma on things surrounding them and struggle to understand events happening around them.

STUCK IN TRAUMA

As the number of psychiatrists remained minimal and veterans were on a constant increase; many veterans weren't attended to, the rate of suicide climbed and the violence rate spiked.

Bessel later started a group for young Vietnam veterans to cushion the effect the war has created in the minds of those affected and discovered that veterans are only comfortable to open up about their true hurt to fellow soldiers. This is because they believe they are the ones that can relate to what they have gone through. It is either you are one of them or you are out of their circle and lose the privilege of hearing their experience on the battlefield. That is why they end up shoving their family away and only warm-up to fellow soldiers.

DIAGNOSING POSTTRAUMATIC STRESS

A tiny factor for veteran's trauma can be attributed to depression, alcoholism, depression, drug abuse, mood malady, etc. But like said earlier, that's just an insignificant fraction of the real issue. As time went on, Bessel registered failure in attempting to solve the trauma of these soldiers. But later in

1980 change came when a new diagnosis called posttraumatic stress disorder (PTSD) by some Vietnam veterans and assisted by Robert J. Lifton and New York psychoanalysts cajoled the American Psychiatric Association on the aforementioned study. This diagnosis helped to group the symptoms associated with fellow veterans. This now helped to understand patients with PTSD better and the solution in sight.

A NEW UNDERSTANDING

From the diagnosis in the past, Bessel concluded that brain imaging gears help to know what hurt his patients, how hurt they are, and how to help. This way, one can interpret how our feelings affect the physical. Trauma doesn't remain in the past which it should, it is the colophon of the event on the human brain, mind, and body.

- **Lessons**
  1. Trauma is not limited to the mind alone, it manifests physiologically.
  2. Trauma is a prison inflicted by Self or another individual that ends up destroying its host.
  3. Group therapy is a ground for healing and learning.
- **Issues surrounding the subject matter**
  1. What traumatic experience are you reliving daily?

  _____

  _____

  _____

  _____

  _____

  2. Why do survivors refuse to let go of past pain?

_____

_____

_____

_____

_____

3. Is it possible to let go of the horrific past, embrace a purposeful future and how do we go about this?

_____

_____

_____

_____

_____

4. Would you agree that categorizing trauma (PTSD) brought a solution and why whether yes or no?

_____

_____

_____

_____

_____

- **Goals**

1. In what ways can traumatized victims regain control of their lives with all the help available to them?

_____

_____

_____

_____

_____

2. In what ways have you received help to extinguish your trauma from hunting you and how did you go about it step by step?

_____
_____
_____
_____
_____
_____
_____
_____
_____
_____
_____
_____
_____
_____

- **Action steps**
  1. Reach out to someone that can help, don't be silent about all you are battling inside
- **Checklist**
  1. Trauma isn't the end of the world; you can find yourself again.

CHAPTER 2: REVOLUTIONS IN UNDERSTANDING MIND AND BRAIN

Bessel stumbled upon the execution of a research during his time in medical school in 1960 in the Massachusetts Mental Health Center to determine the most appropriate way to cure young people that suffered their initial mental breakdown identified as "schizophrenia".

In 1950, some French scientists came together to find a new compound called – chlorpromazine sold as Thorazine. This drug tackled symptoms of schizophrenia such as anxiety, depression, panic, and helped to relax patients making them calm and less delusional.

TRAUMA BEFORE DAWN

Bessel, a young doctor at the time resided in the psychiatry unit and realized that patients found it hard to sleep, so they come out to talk. He noticed that during this time of peace, the patients reveal a lot that caused them to be in their present state. He concluded that those midnight revelations are very relevant in discovering how damaged the patient is, the true cause of the trauma, and how to help them out of it. His findings revealed that over half of the patients in a psychiatric home are victims of assault, neglect, witnesses to violence, or physical abuse.

He couldn't help but notice the detached manner in which doctors reported patients' symptoms or the poor enthusiasm to help them discover the possible cure for their debilitating and degrading mental state. Bessel discovered a thesis in Eugen Bleuler's textbook on "Dementia Praecox" which revealed something rather intriguing about schizophrenic body hallucinations. He mentioned that sexual hallucinations are the most vital and frequent. Patients hallucinate of the most bizarre kind of sexual satisfaction from their well of sexual fantasy. It is more fascinating they admit to feeling real sensations. Now, does this go to say that people can only hallucinate over an image they had experienced? Are they fragments of a real-life experience they are reliving? How thin is the line between being creative and a pathological imagination?

Traumatized people lack coordination and precision. They are with little or no emotion and carry on conversations very stiff.

MAKING SENSE OF SUFFERING

Bessel's teacher Elvin Semrad at MMHC pointed out that the ultimate of human suffering is related to loss and love. Humans suffer much when they lie to themselves. He admonished them as therapists to tell patients the truth about the harsh reality of life. Therapists are to help suffering patients come to terms with the way the world works and help them bear this reality. Survivors can begin to recover when they know what they truly feel, can interpret that feeling and a possible solution will be administered. The result of a study that brought a new wave for tackling psychological challenges was published in the American

Journal of Psychiatry in 1968 which revealed that schizophrenic patients treated with drugs only came out better than those who spoke therapeutically with the best of therapists at the time in Boston.

The 19th century sprang up the need to examine behavior as an alteration to the difficulties of this world such as pride, sloth, anger, greed, lust, and any other disorder that falls in the category. Antipsychotic drugs became a respite for the long years of increasing numbers of psychiatric patients. Bessel's success story with an antipsychotic drug – Lithium he administered to a woman having recurring insanity returned with tremendous testimonies. Soon afterward, as medication for the subject matter increased, so did more patients that had been confined and chained with no breakthrough in their treatment began to record success.

In 1960, the National Institutes of Health scientists discovered the need to study and develop ways of separating and rationalizing hormones and neurotransmitters in the brain and blood. This was to help develop drugs that will address a specific abnormality in the brain due to the irregular levels of norepinephrine connected to depression and dopamine using schizophrenia. But that didn't go very far and the same did the *Diagnostic and Statistical Manual of Mental Disorders* (DSM), known as the "bible of psychiatry.

INESCAPABLE SHOCK

At this point, it appeared that neuroscience could answer Bessel's many questions relating to traumatic stress. A lecture by Steven Maier of the University of Colorado aided by Martin

Seligman of the University of Pennsylvania was carried out on animals; dogs specifically. The act required administering electric shocks to dogs that have been locked up in cages for long; a condition called "inescapable shock".

The result of the research revealed that the dogs that were administrated inescapable shock didn't run off when the cages were open except those that weren't shocked. This explains that the traumatized tend to build a wall around themselves and stay in its confines when their stress hormones are elevated. They are seemingly comfortable in their entitled fear and easily give up. The fate faced by the dogs is similar to that of the patients which receive a shock in therapy to soothe their trauma. It's either the patient's agitation is heightened or it leads to a terrible breakdown.

The dogs that experienced the fight, flight, and freeze signals long after the shock occurred had to be dragged out of their cage to show them what freedom looks like. So, does it mean that the same technique applies to humans in other to gain back control over their lives? Can they be taught to defend themselves in hazardous and life-threatening situations that lead to traumatic experiences?

ADDICTED TO TRAUMA: THE PAIN OF PLEASURE AND THE PLEASURE OF PAIN

In the act of confessing and relating everything they have gone through, they significantly brighten up in their debilitating mental state and horrific stories. Traumatized people feel empty and unfulfilled when they are not stressed, nervous, angry, and in a life-threatening situation. They chase experiences that a normal mind will rationally evade. They have a strong compulsion to repeat the same event that has put them in their bad state.

Findings by Richard Solomon of the University of Pennsylvania revealed that the human body bends to various kinds of stimuli. That's why what will ordinarily cause pain and discomfort such as parachute jumping, or marathon race will be a pleasurable experience to others due to the change in the chemical balance of the body.

In 1946, a publication named – "Pain in Men Wounded in Battle" revealed that a measure of increased emotions can block the sensation of pain. This was evident that 75% of gravely wounded soldiers refused morphine to ease their pain. It was discovered also that the pain they felt released morphine-like substances in their blood.

SOOTHING THE BRAIN

A finding by Professor Jeffrey Gray of Kings College shows that serotonin reduces the liability to get easily stressed. It revealed that animals with serotonin levels knew nothing about handling stress, thus they freeze or get aggressive. Serotonin was found to help in handling potentially threatening situations and reduce their fear level. The question now is; can serotonin help PTSD patients since it helps to improve the functionality of the brain? Later in 1988, the 8th of February to be precise, a drug called Prozac of fluoxetine was introduced for trauma-related patients. Prozac brought tremendous change to the traumatized folks. Many began to reason more articulately and slept better. But, Prozac didn't change the PTSD state of the war veterans.

THE TRIUMPH OF PHARMACOLOGY

Pharmacology enabled psychiatry to evolve. Drugs were introduced as a tool aside from normal therapy sessions. This empowerment became a source of income for psychiatric Doctors and they made an immense profit. Abandoned buildings were converted for the use of psychiatric treatments as progress with traumatized patients were maintained.

With this good news, bad news still lurks around. The entrance of medications that aids sanity in people also led to the high consumption of antidepressants today. As the numbers keep climbing (medical report on consumption explains so) fewer people go in for proper therapy, instead, they rely on stronger antidepressants like Risperdal, Abilify, Seroquel, and Zyprexa which has a strong downside. Shouldn't these doctors that are prescribing these drugs be held accountable? Don't get me wrong, drugs are needed but encouraging and the abuse of it can pose a more traumatic position.

- **Lessons**
  1. Traumatized people feel empty and unfulfilled when they are not stressed, nervous, angry, and in a life-threatening situation.
  2. Inescapable shock technique is no solution to ending the trauma demons from attacking its victim.
  3. Doctors don't pay much attention to patients addicted to antidepressants. Thus the increase that addiction.
  4. The introduction of medicine in psychiatry revolutionized it.
- **Issues surrounding the subject matter**

1. Shouldn't these doctors that are prescribing these drugs be held accountable?

_____

_____

_____

_____

2. Is human suffering only related to loss and love and why?

_____

_____

_____

_____

3. Why do humans lie to themselves when it only leads to more suffering?

_____

_____

_____

_____

4. Is it true that people can only hallucinate over an image they had experienced?

_____

_____

_____

_____

5. How thin is the line between being creative and a pathological imagination?

_____

_____

_____

_____

_____

- **Goals**
  1. In what ways can doctors help patients from being addicted to trauma-related drugs?

  _____

  _____

  _____

  _____

  _____

  _____

  _____

  _____

  _____

  2. It was noticed that talking about the horrific experience helped most of the patients live life again, how do you intend to apply the same technique to help trauma suffering individuals and if you are a past traumatized person; what techniques were adopted that helped you?

  _____

  _____

  _____

  _____

  _____

  _____

_____

_____

_____

_____

_____

_____

_____

_____

_____

- **Action steps**
  1. As a therapist, tell patients the truth about the harsh reality of life so they can grow a tough skin.
  2. How you treat psychiatric patient matters, try not to replicate their past with your method of care.
- **Checklist**
  1. Understanding how the mind and brain work following the traumatized can reveal the extent to which they are affected and how to help.

CHAPTER 3
LOOKING INTO THE BRAIN: THE NEUROSCIENCE REVOLUTION

Brain-visualizing practices of the 1990's paved way for possible ways to comprehend the different ways the human brain functions and process information. Neuroscience gained ground with the creation of colossal and pricy machines on computer technology and advanced physics such as functional magnetic resonance imaging (fMRI) and positron emission (PET) that allowed scientists proper imagery of the activities going on in the brain parts.

With this new understanding in mind, neuroscience gave a better meaning to trauma on all grounds. Later in 1994, Scott Rauch, the first director of the Massachusetts General Hospital Neuroimaging Laboratory researched eight patients using images, memories, and sounds associated with the past event to discover which part of the brain is stimulated during danger, why, and to what extent. It was discovered that the limbic area of the brain was the most responsive part which holds the amygdala. This part is responsible for warnings on imminent danger and stimulates the appropriate stress reaction.

SPEECHLESS HORROR

The Broca's part of the brain is one of the centers responsible for speech. A decline in that area will lead to loss of proper processing of thoughts and will be impossible to relate it in words – This is peculiar in traumatized people when they relive experiences that trigger anger, terror, defenselessness, and the strong desire to flee or fight.

SHIFTING TO ONE SIDE OF THE BRAIN

Scan reports have it that flashbacks ignite the right side of the brain popularly stereotyped to be responsible for the emotional, artistic, and intuitive display in humans.

The left side of the brain is analytical, verbal, orderly. It recalls statistics and facts to the latter while the right side of the brain keeps memoirs of smell, emotions, sound, and touch. The right side of the brain first develops in the womb; that's what enables the mother and fetus to communicate. With the peculiarities of different halves of the brain carrying out distinct functions, it is incapacitating for one half to function in isolation of the other. When flashbacks happen to traumatized people, the right side of the brain is triggered and they become afraid, angry, ashamed, and withdrawn. Shutting down the left part which would have told them that they are not re-experiencing the past but it's only a rude recall of what the memory holds.

STUCK IN FIGHT OR FLIGHT

One of the hormones crucial to help fight/flee/freeze when faced with harsh situations is adrenaline. Increased heart rate and blood pressure are attributed to a spike in adrenaline. For normal people when there is a spike in adrenaline due to events that call for the increase; after the danger is averted, the body system returns to normal. But in the case of traumatized people, very little things in the direction of the past increases their stress hormones and it takes unreasonably too long to normalize.

The result of constantly increased stress hormones leads to bad temper, retention and attention complications, sleep disorders, and various lasting health issues. This stress also affected the physical body and not only the brain. As the muscles of the body stretch and stiffens whether for fight or flight mode, it negatively affects various parts of the body organ. So we can conclude that the human body sure records each score.

- **Lessons**
  1. One of the hormones crucial to help fight/flee when faced with harsh situations is adrenaline.
  2. The left side of the brain is analytical, verbal, orderly. It recalls statistics and facts to the latter while the right side of the brain keeps memoirs of smell, emotions, sound, and touch.
  3. The traumatized are stuck in the past, they struggle endlessly to be in the present.
- **Issues surrounding the subject matter**
  1. What happens in cases where one side of the brain is only functioning, can an orientation/medication help to restore it to the status quo?

  _____

  _____

  _____

  _____

  _____

- **Goals**
  1. How can traumatized people learn to control their stress hormone and stop overreacting?

  _____

  _____

  _____

  _____

  _____

- **Action steps**
    1. Find a way not to be stuck in the freeze, flight, or fight mode for unnecessarily long.
- **Checklist**
    1. A traumatized person's incapacitated state doesn't just occur overnight, it builds over time.

Bessel used a real-life event of the World Trade Center bombing to explain the role parents play in constructing emotions appropriately from a tender age. A 5-year-old child who witnessed the bombing from his classroom window was able to shake it off and move on because he saw how calm and collected his family managed the situation.

Instead of a psychological scar left behind in the 5-year-old child, he drew the event of the bombing but with a trampoline at the foot of the building. His imagination was able to be rational enough to proffer a solution to the people that jumped out the building's window; but unfortunately to the victims, the trampoline only exists in the drawing. The moral of the story is how his mind played an adaptive role; he fled the site to evade danger and went home. When he was totally out of harm's way, he quickly adjusted to the fact that the threat is over and life can return to normal. Unlike traumatized people, they get stuck in that event and relive it every day – they let no new experience in and get trapped in the past.

ORGANIZED TO SURVIVE

When the oldest part of the brain comes alive, it partially turns off the greater brain which enables the body to either run, freeze, hide, or fight. The old part of the brain takes total control of the body and one of the aforementioned characteristics takes place, as soon as the threat is over, the body returns to its former status. But in cases where the victim is stuck and the supposed response is obstructed, as in cases of rape and kidnap; the stress chemicals keep emitting wastefully in the brain – that even long after the danger is over, the brain still senses danger and the physical body aims to escape.

Going deeper into neuroscience reveals that the brain works interconnected with other parts of the body with the sole aim of helping humans have the best of wellbeing and survive at all costs in the presence of imminent traumatic experiences.

THE BRAIN FROM BOTTOM TO TOP

The brain has a crucial duty to perform and that is to ensure the host survives regardless of the situation. For this to be successful, the brain disseminates indicators syncing with what the body needs per time like; shelter, food, sex, food, security, and more. As mammals functioned to follow what our internal organs propose, it becomes a grave challenge when the internal organs stop working. Trauma is lethal and it disrupts the functionality of the brain.

The human brain is built gradually from birth (called reptilian brain which is responsible for every stable internal equilibrium in the infant known as homeostasis), with the cognitive brain being the youngest part occupying just 30% of the internal part of the skull. This part of the brain figures out how you can achieve your goals and aspirations, give order to your actions and help in the proper management of your time. Underneath this part is two older but different parts of the brain that takes care of the safety of the body, fatigue, lust, pain, threat, comfort, hunger, joy, and even pleasure. Anything that alters the normal sensation one should feel as a human is a serious cause for concern.

The limbic system known as the mammalian brain lays immediately above the reptilian brain. Infants learn of the world by everything they do, smiling, what triggers them to cry, crawl, move, and even to object when addressed.

For the frontal lobes, there is the neocortex which is the top part of the brain we share with other mammals. This part develops quickly as it assumes the 2nd year of its life. These lobes are accountable for what makes humans distinct in the animal kingdom, makes us constructive to use words to communicate instead of being limited to using only gestures, helps in better planning, reflection, and imagination.

MIRRORING EACH OTHER: INTERPERSONAL NEUROBIOLOGY

Mirror neurons were discovered by some Italian scientists in 1994 within specialized cells in the cortex. Using monkeys, the researcher put electrodes specific to each neuron in the monkey's premotor region and track which neuron ignited when the monkey was actively picking objects before him. As this went on, the pseudoscientist kept placing food bits inside a box, as he watched the computer; the monkey's brain cells lighted up in the exact region the motorized command neurons resided. This goes to emphasize that the mirror neurons are capable of imitating, synchronization, compassion, and even initiate the growth of a language.

IDENTIFYING DANGER: THE COOK & THE SMOKE DETECTOR

The area of the brain referred to as the "cook" is the thalamus. This part is responsible for sending several sensations of what the body is experiencing and sends them to the amygdala and to the frontal lobes where we become aware of the situation. This has the typical trait of a smoke detector helping the host take cover or flee. In times when the thalamus crashes, natural sensations like touch, sound, smell, and sight are processed individually, and time halts and makes a present danger take forever.

CONTROLLING THE STRESS RESPONSE: THE WATCHTOWER

As the amygdala serves as a sure smoke detector, the medial prefrontal cortex (MPFC) above the eyes serves as a watchtower to make sure what the amygdala is reacting accordingly – fight, flight, or just smokescreen. This balance is necessary to help your system put some checks and balances to the signal from the amygdala. But, in a traumatized person's case (increased sadness, rage, and fear), the amygdala and the MPFC are difficult to control due to the surge in the subcortical part of the brain which was stimulated.

THE RIDER AND THE HORSE

Emotions and reason are not so different from the other. Our emotions give value to events and serve as the base of our reasoning. When our rational and emotional brains are threatened and survival is dicey, the aforementioned will be forced to work in isolation of the other.

A neuroscientist, Paul Maclean explained the relationship between the emotional brain and the rational brain as that of an incompetent rider and his disobedient/wild horse. A serene and smooth road will make both the rider and the horse go seamlessly; but immediately distractions erupt like sounds and movement from other animals, the horse becomes uneasy and the rider latches on top the horse with every fiber in his being.

The same happens when people feel their survival is threatened, they can't reason any more.

- **Lessons**
  1. Neuroscience reveals that the brain works interconnected with other parts of the body with the sole aim of helping humans have the best of wellbeing and survive at all costs in the presence of imminent traumatic experiences.
  2. Mirror neurons are capable of imitating, synchronization, compassion, and even initiate the growth of a language.
- **Issues surrounding the subject matter**
  1. Is it possible to live in the present when the past haunts you day and night?

  _____

  _____

  _____

  _____

  _____

  2. What is responsible for being stuck in the past even when in the present?

  _____

  _____

  _____

  _____

  _____

  _____

- **Goals**

1. What do you understand by the anatomy of survival and how can one live above a traumatized state?

_____

_____

_____

_____

_____

_____

_____

_____

_____

_____

- **Action steps**
  1. The brain has a crucial duty to perform and that is to ensure the host survives regardless of the situation. You help out by giving a helping hand.
- **Checklist**
  1. Comprehending the disparity between the top and bottom functionality of the brain is fundamental to knowing and solving traumatic stress.

Charles Darwin's *"Expression of the Emotions in Man and Animals"* in 1872 exposed fundamental insights to the foundations of the emotional life of humans, packed with annotations and narratives culled from eras of investigation, alongside tales of Darwin's children and pets at home.

Darwin posits in his book that all mammals have equal emotions, senses, passions, affections, intuition, and even the same physical characteristics. He oddly referred to humans as just mere "Men" while he called animals "Higher animals" — maybe he is biased because he is an animal lover.

His likening humans to animals' point of view is stated in his book as he says humans get frightened and the hairs at the back of their necks stand just like animals, we feel angry and clench of teeth in rage just the way animals do. Darwin says — it has everything to do with biology and evolution. Darwin's interconnectedness with mammals and the way humans function is explained in his position on PTSD. It says that when the human mind is trapped in survival mode, they lose track of more important things like care, love, family, affection, growth, nurture, learning, play, and kill everything around them.

A WINDOW INTO THE NERVOUS SYSTEM

All the body parts work interconnected to the other as a distinct regulatory system. The synchronization of the body system is attributed to both divisions of the autonomic nervous system (ANS) — the sympathetic and the parasympathetic. When the former helps in accelerating the body (arousal, fight and flight reaction and triggers the gland responsible for disseminating adrenaline); the latter works as its brake and encourages some self-conserving qualities like; digestion and injury healing.

The Polyvagal Theory opened our eyes more to a clearer understanding of biology and how it relates to safety and danger

THE NEURAL LOVE CODE

The Polyvagal Theory opened our eyes more to a clearer understanding of biology and how it relates to safety and danger. It looks far beyond the backlash of fight and flight and gave more cognizance to social relationships at the forefront and our comprehension of trauma at the core. We are built for connection and not isolation. When this natural functionality is defied, then we begin to struggle.

SAFETY AND RECIPROCITY

Attaining safety amongst fellow humans is a healthy attribute and a walk in the right direction. This way, you are assured of a significant and substantial life. For traumatized people, they only connect among fellow traumatized patients with similar dark experiences and they have a sense of belonging even if reliving the traumatic experience will bring more pain.

THREE LEVELS OF SAFETY

Several events in life determine which survival mode we assume and which we don't attempt depending on the case study. These 3 levels of safety are; social engagement, flight or fight, and freeze or collapse. Every experience the brain gains shapes it. Humans stay humans by bonding together with fellow humans, take care of their children, be responsible for their immediate families, and the society at large, and defend their loved ones in times of danger. For most traumatized people, the root cause or base of their trauma experience is immobilization. The question is, when does one defend themselves or just let fate take its course? The normal pattern of the brain is to always be on alert but in other to accommodate another person's love, we switch off our defense and lay down our guard. On the other side of the divide, traumatized people are always hypervigilant to enjoy the life that the present offers while some others are very disoriented to let in any new experience.

- **Lessons**
  1. The human body registers the score.
  2. The memory of trauma is programmed in the viscera, heartbreaking emotions, automobile disorders, and muscular/skeletal difficulties, making emotion parameter a crucial need in therapeutic expectations.
- **Issues surrounding the subject matter**
  1. Asides emotion is a yardstick to evaluate trauma, what other components are necessary to make this work?

  _____

  _____

  _____

  _____

  _____

- **Goals**
  1. How can a traumatized person in flight/fight mode be disengaged?

  _____

  _____

_____

_____

2. What is your take on tapping into social engagement and making traumatized patients active to relieve them of their pain?

_____

_____

_____

_____

3. How can our educational system infuse the emotional-engagement into treating the traumatized?

_____

_____

_____

_____

_____

- **Action steps**
  1. Don't respond in an irritated manner to the traumatized, especially if you are doing everything within your might to find a solution.
- **Checklist**
  1. There are 3 levels of safety; social engagement, flight or fight, and freeze or collapse

The human composite is capable of sensing objects based on their shape, weight, feel, and even temperature with our eyes closed. When this isn't happening, that's to say our sensory perception is dead – this is most common with people with PTSD having clogged senses.

Dr. Ruth Lanius revealed how trauma affects self-awareness with concerns with sensory self-awareness. Her research was on individuals with childhood abuse which had to lay in a brain scanner to ascertain what happens in the brain when no thought is running to and fro in it. The result was fascinating, the brain's concentration on "self" increased. When the brain isn't thinking and roaming about, its entire energy is directed to self. Discovering "Self" which is self-awareness is a big step in the right direction if we are to find solutions to trauma. It begins from the frontal part of the brain which comprises of the medial prefrontal cortex, the orbital prefrontal cortex, the insula, the anterior cingulate, and the posterior cingulate. In the cases of severely traumatized people, they have successfully cut off that area in the brain (medial prefrontal activation) that makes them susceptible to feelings and emotions. This makes them live without purpose, direction, and ultimately self-awareness.

Damasio from a minute think tank meeting explained our sensory world came to be before we were conceived. His stand on the relationship among emotions, the body, and survival is clear – the mind is capable of not only finding facts but to also hide them. The body is like a screen that hides the interior perfectly well. The backlash is that while one is busy attending to physical things in the day, the origin of "Self" will be abated. As the brain constantly monitors and evaluates the happenings of the interior and exterior environment, our conscious self needs to unwaveringly keep our internal stability by acting on our physical feelings to help in keeping our bodies safe, away from the threat, groom yourself to take ownership of your own life, befriend your body and cease seeing yourself as a stranger or separate from your body (depersonalization); lastly and very important – connect with others if you are finding yourself once again.

- **Lessons**
  1. People with trauma struggle to recognize what is going on in their bodies.
  2. Neglect and severe emotional abuse are the same as sexual molestation and physical abuse.
- **Issues surrounding the subject matter**
  1. If it is true that what goes on inside our brains determines how we feel, and that our body feelings are coordinated by subconscious brain structures, how can we gain control over them?

_____
_____
_____
_____
_____
_____
_____
_____

2. In your opinion, do you think PTSD patients should trust their therapists with their deepest secrets & why?

_____

_____

_____

_____

_____

- **Goals**
  1. How do you think traumatized people can acquire and incorporate common sensory understanding so that they can live life naturally giving the appropriate responses to touch and feeling and also feel safe and whole in their bodies?

  _____

  _____

  _____

  _____

  _____

  2. How can people with PTSD take back control of their brain when trapped in a fight for survival?

  _____

  _____

  _____

  _____

  _____

  _____

  _____

  _____

- **Action steps**
  1. A popular response to pain is to reach out to people we love and trust to help us and give us the courage we need to move on.
  2. Encourage them to join activities that will involve social synchronization, it helps to build back their self-confidence and worth.
- **Checklist**
  1. People with trauma need to open up their hearts to get a tangible result from therapy sessions.

CHAPTER 7

GETTING ON THE SAME WAVELENGTH: ATTACHMENT AND ATTUNEMENT

Bessel with the help of his colleague Nina Fish-Murray brought together a set of test cards for the disturbed and disturbing children of "The Children's Clinic" at the Massachusetts Mental Health Center (MMHC) using image cutlets from magazines. The test was done on 12 children from MMHC and a school close by from ages 6 -11 based on their race, age, family group, and intelligence.

The result of the test which differentiated the hospitalized kids from the kids in the control group was the evidence of abuse from their families. The control group which was of poor children and resided in violence-prone areas, nevertheless when presented an image illustrating a family scene of two kids smiling as they watched their father repair their family car; the hospitalized children saw the only danger as the father laid beneath the car, another child saw how one of the kids was going to smash the father in the head with a hammer, or that the children in the image will kick away the jack so the car is suspended on the father beneath with lots of blood on the garage floor, but in the case of the control kids – they said the car will be fixed and the family will go for a fun outing in it.

After showing several other images to both groups, it was clear that the kids in the control group still had faith and see the world as a kind and beautiful place even if they live in an area that perpetuates crime and violence; but the hospitalized kids had long ago thrown in the towel and given up on anything good about life and all they can see and sense is rage, inappropriate sexual urge, fear and exaggerated danger due to their history of constant abuse.

There are several other factors attributed to the upbringing that is responsible for the insanity experienced by traumatized persons such as the lag in motherly care especially for men taken early from their mother's arms which is responsible for their misbehavior. Separating a young child from its mother has a way of affecting the child's psyche and ultimately hinders the discovery of "Self".

As social beings, we seek to be amongst a homogenous community actively impacting one another in the little way possible. We begin to learn from the time we are born, with every care we receive, we learn how to dote on ourselves and care for others. A peaceful and loving home will most times nurture a confident, self-reliant, and emphatic child.

During this time, all the love, care, and attention given to the child make a secure connection (bond) with both mother and child. Children who acquire a strong connection from a tender age know how others feel when they feel bad, they know what makes one feels good and they also know to alter the way they feel and other people's feedback.

Children naturally attach. They always want to be with their parents or caregivers regardless of how insensitive, abusive or neglecting they may be. But, these seemingly unresponsive kids only show their excessive arousal in their persistent increased heart rate. They detest touch, they don't trust anyone, they sense danger all times because they lack an internal sense of safety and can't differentiate the latter with danger, they are disorganized (one moment they want to be held and the next moment they fight to be free being held or cuddled), – called "disorganized attachment".

THE LONG-TERM EFFECTS OF DISORGANIZED ATTACHMENT

Disorganized attachment's long-term effects are; role reversal (mother wanting love from the child), emotional distancing, neglect, hostile, insensitive, fearful, etc. That's why it's no surprise that a mother will abuse her child. These children then tend to grow up unstable and without a sense of self having traits of; promiscuity, drug abuse, reckless, wasteful spending, suicidal, and enhanced anger. Harmony must be restored to our lives to help us overcome challenges and detachment even in the face of distress and frustration without falling into trauma.

- **Lessons**
  1. We are social beings and we seek to amongst a homogenous community.
  2. As the physical connection is necessary for the discovery of Self; the kinesthetic and visceral sensation of how our bodies meet is what makes it all real.
- **Issues surrounding the subject matter**
  1. Can the effects of disorganized attachment be avoided from childhood till adulthood and how?

_____

_____

_____

_____

_____

- **Goals**

1. How possible is it to reframe the mind and brain of abused children?

_____

_____

_____

_____

_____

2. How can one get to enable the trust and confidence of brutalized children that have known only pain from a tender age?

_____

_____

_____

_____

_____

_____

_____

_____

_____

- **Action steps**
    1. Harmony is to be restored in other to overcome challenges.
- **Checklist**
    1. A peaceful and loving home will most times nurture a confident, self-reliant, and emphatic child.

CHAPTER 8

TRAPPED IN RELATIONSHIPS: THE COST OF ABUSE AND NEGLECT

It is one thing to be traumatized and another thing to discover the truth behind the symptoms you possess. Symptoms like a compulsive urge to throw up any meal eaten, cutting oneself with a blade to reduce numbness, etc. It is of utmost importance for patients to learn ways of tolerating their feeling and identify what they know.

It is very hard for traumatized patients to differentiate between what is safe and what isn't; what should be repelled and what should be embraced. Like mentioned before, the foundation of anything matters a lot. A child who grew up with love, adoration, and care will recognize the opposite immediately it shows up. This treatment will repel as unfamiliar and crude. But in the case of children that are accustomed to abuse, they witness to the hostility and neglect as a normal part of life and that singular orientation shapes their life on the relationship, association, and more.

As a therapist, your job is not to stop traumatized patients from feeling sorrow for themselves or blaming them but to assist in restructuring their inner map of how they perceive the world. As an adult, it's not too late to learn to love, trust and feel again – the fact that you were abused and neglected doesn't make everyone else in the world a monster no matter how many times you tried. Some techniques can help trauma patients let go of what they have heavy inside such as; remembering the ordeal intentionally and calmly – pay attention to your breathing, six breaths a minute deeply in and out accompanying the feelings of the breath of your body. Gain total control of your physical sensation by keeping your mind alive and feel the sensations that drowned you slowly purposefully. The idea is that you control the way you feel, your thoughts, and the length at which you allow the thoughts of the ordeal showcase in the mind.

Therapists need to give more time to patients to divulge their past at their own pace, it's more effective and result-driven. Forcing them will drive them more into eliminating awareness and build a fortress around self-denial at their lethal detriment.

- **Lessons**
    1. Victims of incest have trouble differentiating between danger and safety.
    2. A typical but scary reality of child sexual abuse hinges on isolation, Initiation, helplessness, intimidation, self-blame, and stigmatization.
- **Issues surrounding the subject matter**
    1. As a therapist, it is advisable to push or inquire of your patients every horrid detail of their past?

    _____

    _____

    _____

    _____

    _____

- **Goals**
    1. What kind of method should be applied and in what ways should patients with trauma be handled in other for them to open up about their experience so that help can come for them?

_____

_____

_____

_____

_____

_____

_____

_____

_____

_____

- **Action steps**
  1. As parents, guardians, and therapist, stop watering down experiences related to you by the traumatized. Stop the rejection and hostility and investigate the story before throwing it in the trash.
- **Checklist**
  1. Change can only begin as we learn to embrace our emotional brains.

CHAPTER 9
WHAT'S LOVE GOT TO DO WITH IT?

Assisting someone with trauma to unify their thought pattern largely depends on how their problems are defined, the specific diagnosis for their symptoms, and the available care displayed. Sometimes patients are given a diagnosis that has nothing to do with their symptoms and even given unrelated drugs as well.

Psychiatry is complex because it requires an understanding of what is wrong with people and why they act the way they do. Any subject matter that involves the human mind is highly sensitive. An attempt to make a working psychiatric diagnosis manual happened in 1980 by the American Psychiatric Association (APA) called *Diagnostic and Statistical Manual of Mental Disorders.* Today the American Psychiatric Association has made well above $100 million as a result, but the question is; are these patients getting the solution they desire?

Giving the wrong medication and diagnosis to a trauma patient is lethal and can make the matter worse than it already is. As a therapist, try not to work with diagnostic labels (such as PTSD, bipolar, borderline personality disorder (BPD), etc.). It has a way of framing the patient to believing that is what he is and that's all he will become.

In other to ascertain levels of trauma, its imperative that you take their mark into cognizance. For example, BPD is characterized by dangerous mood swings, extremely unstable relationships, and self-destructive behavior such as countless suicide attempts and self-mutilation. This leads to the need to know the connection between BPD and childhood trauma. It was revealed by Bessel, Judy, and Chris Perry the then director of research in Cambridge Hospital that the symptoms BPD patients display initially started as ways to deal with devastating emotions and inevitable brutality. Secondly, it was concluded that one can never understand BPD without understanding the language of abuse and trauma. It also revealed that most of BPD patients suffered the severe case of neglect/child abuse and its impact is largely dependent on the age it started to occur.

When a child is angry or afraid about been abandoned whether it comes as a threat or not, they are honest about their reaction and it has a lot to do with their experience. When these children have to deny strong experiences they have had, it creates lingering distrust, reverse curiosity, disbelief of their senses and nothing seems real.

The place of diagnosis cannot be downplayed. Today many patients are diagnosed with trauma types that have got nothing to do with them and some that don't even exist at all. If a diagnosis isn't accurate then it's good as nothing because without a proper diagnosis – treatment cannot follow. This poses a grave dilemma for therapists. The concerns of neglect and child abuse are more complex and it supersedes the impact of even natural disasters like hurricanes.

Internist Vincent Felitti discovered in 1985 that most obese patients suffered sexual abuse in time past as children. It further revealed that traumatic life experiences during childhood and adolescence are very common no wonder the children have suicidal tendencies, extreme anger, and distrust. For most adults, they often are in debt, increased workplace absenteeism, lower life wages, practice habits like excessive smoking and drinking, multiple sexual partners, unwanted pregnancies, major health challenges such as chronic obstructive pulmonary disease (COPD), liver disease, and ischemic heart disease.

Identifying the problem is a solution. When a diagnosis is done right and the patient's symptoms match with what is diagnosed it has given the solution a sure direction and possible solution. At other times, the problems can just happen to be the solution. Back to child abuse, this is a great concern in our world today which needs addressing. Enough of allowing children to grow up traumatized and without direction in life, unable to feel pleasure, unable to grow emotionally and academically.

- **Lessons**
  1. Giving the wrong medication and diagnosis to a trauma patient is lethal and can make the matter worse than it already is.
  2. Internist Vincent Felitti discovered in 1985 that most obese patients suffered sexual abuse in time past as children.
  3. When a child is angry or afraid about been abandoned whether it comes as a threat or not, they are honest about their reaction and it has a lot to do with their experience.
- **Issues surrounding the subject matter**
  1. Have you ever been diagnosed wrongly before, how was the outcome and how did you come out of it?

  _____
  _____
  _____

_____

_____

- **Goals**
  1. In your honest opinion and vast experience, what kind of therapies do you feel is effective for people with a history of abuse, predominantly those who feel constantly suicidal and intentionally hurt themselves?

_____

_____

_____

_____

_____

_____

_____

_____

- **Action steps**
  1. Don't assume that you know the problem facing the trauma patient, conduct a diagnosis, and be accurate in your discovery so that the solution will be effective.
- **Checklist**
  1. Psychiatry is complex because it requires an understanding of what is wrong with people and why they act the way they do.

CHAPTER 10

DEVELOPMENTAL TRAUMA: THE HIDDEN EPIDEMIC

There are countless cases of traumatized children than you know. The public has only availed the statistic which may not be accurate, but the numbers keep rising. It's one thing to diagnose a patient based on what has been reported, but it is far much more another thing to know who the patient is and how they can be helped asides from the symptoms displayed or described.

The therapist needs to look further from just finding solutions to these traumatized children through new drug creation or discovering the gene responsible for their ailment. The ultimate need is to help them live a life above all they have passed through, to live productive lives and save up millions of taxpayer's money for other life-changing feats. There exist bad and perverted parents but no bad gene; so no need ascribing bad parenting to bad genes. Schizophrenia was discovered to be an austere and confusing form of mental illness which can be transferred genetically. But after several years there is no record of stable genetic patterns for schizophrenia. Genes are not static and life experiences can frame a gene by triggering biochemical messages that control it.

Trauma fundamentally affects a developing mind, brain, and learning at large. Childhood trauma is very different from traumatic stress as experienced in adults. As trauma for the subjects is studied there is an urgent need for organizations to be set up to promote both studies of childhood trauma and educating those that deal with traumatized children such as mental health professionals, nurses, teachers, physicians, judges, foster parents, and ministers.

THE POWER OF DIAGNOSIS

PTSD is when an individual is open to a horrific event involving real/threatened death/grave injury or a threat to their physical honor or that of others that leads to extreme fear, defenselessness resulting in various symptoms such as intrusive withdrawal, reliving the experience through flashbacks, nightmares, repetition of the event as if in a trance, and heightened arousal – irritability, hypervigilance, and insomnia.

A diagnosis is a powerful tool in the hands of the therapist, after proper diagnosis, one can be treated aright based on the problems derived from the diagnostic process. Without the traumatic root cause of a problem, various labels that look somewhat alike with the symptoms displayed will be bestowed on the patients, labels like "oppositional defiant disorder" because the child is aggressive and unyielding. Many other labels like that are given to patients that before they get to the age of accountability, they will have many senseless labels and receive medication that will only hurt them the more. A typical example of a manual with a myriad of labels is the *Diagnostic and Statistical Manual of Mental Disorders* that was introduced in May 2013.

Thus, it is of utmost importance to dutifully run diagnosis for effective solutions. Some biological factors are responsible for the constant pumping of stress hormones whether real or imagined threats leading to physical challenges such as headaches, sleep disturbances, oversensitivity to touch or sound, and unexplained pain. They get very agitated and withdrawn that they cannot focus or concentrate. They relieve stress in the most awkward, disdainful, and demeaning manner like; chronic masturbation and self-mutilating acts like hail pulling, biting, burning, hitting the body against objects, cutting to bleed out, etc.

HOW RELATIONSHIPS SHAPE DEVELOPMENT

In 1975 Alan Sroufe discovered that the quality of care a child receives and biological factors are intertwined. It was noticed that the kind of relationship shared by the child and its mother is more productive than the mother's persona, or the child IQ or temperament, nor its response to stress because it doesn't foretell if the child would cultivate grave behavioral problems as a teen. How does a parent instill resilience in their kids? How does the parent react when they fall; do they remain in self-pity or do they bounce back from their adversity?

THE LONG-TERM EFFECTS OF INCEST

These traumatized patients experience the following effect;

- Cognitive effects
- Detachment symptoms
- Depression
- Disturbed sexual growth
- Extreme self-hurt
- Increased rate of obesity
- Lost control over their emotions and can hardly concentrate
- Abnormal stress hormone response
- Early puberty
- Unconnected psychiatric diagnoses
  - **Lessons**

1. PTSD is when an individual is open to a horrific event involving real/threatened death/grave injury or a threat to their physical honor or that of others that leads to extreme fear, defenselessness resulting in various symptoms such as intrusive withdrawal, reliving the experience through flashbacks, nightmares, repetition of the event as if in a trance, and heightened arousal – irritability, hypervigilance, and insomnia.

- **Issues surrounding the subject matter**
  1. As a parent or caregiver, how do you react in adversity?

  _____
  _____
  _____
  _____

  _____

- **Goals**
  1. How can the long term effects of incest or any other sexually related abuse be abated and managed?

  _____
  _____
  _____
  _____
  _____
  _____
  _____
  _____
  _____

  _____

2. How should a parent instill resilience in their kids?

_____

_____

_____

_____

_____

_____

_____

_____

_____

- **Action steps**
  1. Therapists need to look further from just finding solutions to these traumatized children through new drug creation or discovering the gene responsible for their ailment.
- **Checklist**
  1. A diagnosis is a powerful tool in the hands of the therapist, proper diagnosis equally effective solution.

By now you will agree that traumatic memory comes with a lot of complexities. A formerly traumatized person who successfully forgot his pain can all of a sudden start to relive his pain because another victim sprang up out of the blues been exploited by the same perpetrator that rendered him useless in time past.

The mind is fickle indeed, how cruel is it to relive what you conquered. When these memory fragments begin to creep in, all the memory of sexual abuse, neglect, and suffering is activated, followed by disturbing images and severe physical symptoms to run its full course. This is a terrible place to be in, it comes with a full dose of shame and disappointment to realize your past came back to haunt you and it is winning.

As a therapist, aim to help control and tolerate the erratic trauma sensations felt by the patient instead of wasting precious time determining what happened to them. Trauma affects patients differently, it is very normal/common for a traumatized person to lose the memory of the violation episode after it happened only recall them all on a later date in bits till his thought pattern aligns and updates.

NORMAL VERSUS TRAUMATIC MEMORY

For the human mind to remember an event and how accurate it was recalled largely depends on the significance it meant to them personally. It all boils down to arousal. Different people have memories that are tied to smell, people, songs, and even places. Immediately that sensation comes, be it a smell; the thought accompanying the smell starts to display. The mind is framed in a way that allows extraordinary event which doesn't occur daily be retained more than the regulars. Events that are either extremely hurtful and extremely exciting.

Based on the above said, traumatic events are organized as emotional traces (images, sounds, smell, and physical feelings) and fragmented sensory.

UNCOVERING THE SECRETS OF TRAUMA

As medicine was infused in the study of many other aspects of mental problems for a better breakthrough in the 19th century, it's first significant break in mental problem discovery was on hysteria characterized by contraction and paralyzes of the muscles, extreme emotional outburst, and susceptibility to suggestion. Hysteria opened up the floor to discover the mystery behind the mind and body. Renowned pioneers in neurology and psychiatry like Sigmund Freud, Jean-Martin Charcot, and Pierre Janet revealed that trauma is at the source of hysteria especially that of childhood sexual abuse. For one reason or the other, the concern in hysteria was significant in France but widely attributed to the politics of that era.

Pierre Janet revealed that behind every PTSD is extreme emotion/arousal and for every time a sensation relating to the trauma is triggered, the mind can't help but play the tape all over again. There exists a difference between narrative memory and traumatic memory. Traumatic memories are not compressed, they are ignited by precise triggers and simultaneously recall it scanty and excessively. On the other hand, a narrative memory is often social and a story relayed for a purpose. Reenactments are stationary, invariable, mortifying, and often isolated.

Disassociation poses a big problem in trauma, really how can the traumatized learn to live in the present if they keep dwelling in the past? There is a need for an integration of components that concerns the trauma so the brain is aware of what is present and what is past and then begin to live life as such. Though psychoanalysis is obscure today the "talking cure culture" still exists to date.

- **Lessons**
  1. Trauma affects patients differently, it is very normal/common for a traumatized person to lose the memory of the violation episode after it happened only recall them all on a later date in bits till his thought pattern aligns and updates.
- **Issues surrounding the subject matter**
  1. Why does the mind recall intriguing events most and hurtful ones mostly?

_____

_____

_____

_____

_____

- **Goals**
  1. In what ways do you think trauma patients can learn to live in the present and not the past?

_____

_____

_____

_____

_____

- **Action steps**

  1. As a therapist, aim to control and tolerate the erratic trauma sensations felt by the patient instead of wasting precious time determining what happened to them.

- **Checklist**

  1. In-depth details about the trauma event will help to forget the past and move on.

For over a century science has been interested in trauma and that drive has made psychoanalysis gain this much popularity today. With the outbreak of World War in 1914, it left many men with dreadful mysterious medical conditions, strange psychological symptoms, and loss of memory. Using their cases to test the motion pictures technology to film every reaction of these soldiers; today YouTube has candid recordings of their mysterious physical posture, spoken words, scared facial expression, and twitches.

"Shell shock" and "neurasthenia" was diagnosed at the beginning of the war by the British. The former was for treating entitled war veterans and a disability pension; While the latter provided nothing. Nevertheless, whichever option one gets is up to the physician treating. It was later noticed that shell shock heightened compromising the productivity of the combatants who were distracted on whether to bear their pain as soldiers or aim to win the battle over the Germans. Later in June 1917, General Routine Order Number 2384 of the British General Staff stated the term "shell shock" is prohibited to be said verbally or recorded whether casually or in a medical document.

Thus, soldiers with mental problems got a single diagnosis of – Not Yet Diagnosed, Nervous (NYDN). In the face of the abandonment and rejection caused by politics and medicine on returning soldiers, the movie industry and even popular literature relayed the happenings and outcome of the war (just like Hollywood director John Huston's documentary *Let There Be Light* (1946) revealed the hypnosis was the main treatment for war neurosis at the time). The denial of the effects of trauma can destroy the peace of society. This led to militarism and fascism in 1930 leading to the ruthlessness and inhumanity in the Nazi era.

As time went on, trauma took a new face. Using hypnosis as a tool, soldiers were able to express all their deepest fears, worry, pain, survivor's guilt, and differing loyalties. They were able to control their hostility and rage than younger veterans. Doctors help in influencing how their patient responds to pain – when a patient complains of terrible nightmares and the doctor conducts an X-ray on him, that automatically tells him focusing more on his physical problems is far better. Care was administered to these veterans quite alright, but the adoption of intentionally unrecognizing the psychological scars of war killed the traumatic neuroses and erased it from the endorsed psychiatric catalog.

TRAUMA REDISCOVERED

Concerns on traumatic memory loss moved the attention from the atrocity committed to politics and law. Even after Bessel attested with the credible fact that traumatized victims of incest and sexual abuse can tend to forget the painful episode and the recall later when a stimulation ignited it again, lawyers who represented the big dogs (priests, politicians, etc.) said the memory of the victims are just based on False Memory Syndrome meaning that victims fabricated these sequence of sexual abuse and must have been manipulated by their therapist who strives to be relevant at all cost. But that wasn't the case here, then later in the 1980s till early 1990s, victims of one level of sexual and domestic abuse or the other began to find the strength to come out and tell their stories and seek justice led to the framework for the pedophile scandals in the Catholic Church which moved the issue from science to law and politics as memory experts and law experts dragged on in court in the United States and later in Australia and Europe.

THE SCIENCE OF REPRESSED MEMORY

In 1980 the DSM-III acknowledged the presence of memory loss for traumatic events in the diagnostic criteria for dissociative amnesia. Memory loss is a very common phenomenon with victims of childhood sexual abuse. Also, people who suffered from experiences such as accidents, torture, natural disaster, kidnap, war, and other levels of physical abuse.

Dr. Linda Meyer Williams conducted studies on repressed memory using 206 girls within the ages of 10 and 12 years with reported sexual abuse in the early 1970s in Pennsylvania when she was a graduate student of sociology. With documented interviews of them and their parents attesting to the abuse; 17 years after Dr. Linda Meyer Williams tracked down 136 of those girls now adults and conducted an extensive sequel interview to test the strength of their memory as it concerned their past abuse. 38 percent of them didn't remember the abuse, 12 percent refuted ever been abused as a child, 68 percent told other incidents of childhood sexual abuse different from what the record had 17 years ago, 16 percent of the ladies recalled their trauma vividly but confirmed that they forgot some time ago. The younger they are during the incident and the relationship shared with the molester affects the level of memory recall. Once a memory is unreachable; the mind cannot alter it, but as soon as it relayed time and time again it begins to change sequence and content. The meaning we make out of life alters what and how we remember it. Framed memories lack the intuitive reaction expected and the subject gives themselves away in the organization of the memories.

- **Lessons**
  1. Culture shapes the appearance of traumatic stress.
  2. The crux of trauma is unbearable, unbelievable, and overwhelming.
  3. Individual patient impresses on doctors to suspend their realism of what is typical and agree that the patient is dealing with a dual reality: the certainty of a moderately secure and foreseeable present that lives alongside a catastrophic, ubiquitous past.
- **Issues surrounding the subject matter**
  1. Can one recover from the unbearable heaviness of trauma and what ways can that happen?

  _____
  _____
  _____
  _____
  _____

- **Goals**
  1. How do you intend to begin to study the memories of trauma survivors to fully comprehend what goes on in the mind of a traumatized?

  _____
  _____
  _____
  _____

_____

_____

_____

_____

_____

_____

- **Action steps**

  1. To comprehend trauma overcome your usual unwillingness to face that harsh reality and develop the nerve to pay attention to the testimonies of survivors.

- **Checklist**

  1. Unreachable memory cannot be changed.

CHAPTER 13

HEALING FROM TRAUMA: OWNING YOUR SELF

The aftermath of the war, molestation, rape, or any other form of abuse cannot be treated or undone – but what can be done to alleviate the pain and trauma accompanying the event is dealing with the footprints of the trauma on the soul, mind, and body of the victim resulting in nightmares, rage, withdrawal, disassociation and more. By now we all know what trauma steals from us, it takes ownership of our entire being. We cease to exist and the trauma pilots our ship how it wishes till it ruins us.

The main challenge now is to take back ownership of your body, mind, and soul. It takes being aware of your traumatic episode but being in total control of your emotions ranging from; shame, fear, anger, etc. This will involve the following;

- Maintaining a calm posture even abreast of your pain.
- Maintaining a calm and collected posture in response to the sensations that remind you of your past such as images, sounds, thoughts, and even physical sensations.
- Being fully alive in the present and actively engaged socially to your environment and its people.
- Not keeping secrets from yourself and the way you succeeded in surviving your trauma.

A NEW FOCUS FOR RECOVERY

Trauma goes beyond a story about a past event that happened. The trauma imprints resulting in emotions and physical senses disrupts the present state of a person, so it's imperative to regain control of your present by reexamining the trauma all in a bid to confront your fears till you feel safe, then it will never be used as a weapon to traumatize you.

LIMBIC SYSTEM THERAPY

The first step to finding a solution to traumatic stress is by restoring the original balance between the emotional and the rational brains to regain complete control of your life. This involves self-confidence and the ability to be creative and light-hearted. When the mind is extremely aroused or collapses at any given opportunity, it cannot learn anything new talk more of gaining new experiences to quench the impact of the hazardous one that needs to go.

To alter the responses of posttraumatic stress requires gaining access to the emotional brain by conducting a "limbic system therapy". This entails fixing the damaged alarm systems and repairing the emotional brain to the serene place for constructive thinking, safety checks, and takes charge of your general housekeeping, children's safety, and defends against imminent danger.

The emotional brain can be accessed consciously via self-awareness through stimulating the medial prefrontal cortex – the part of the brain that allows us to feel what we are feeling inside of us (technically called "*interoception*" its Latin for – looking inside).

THINGS TO DO TO BEFRIEND THE EMOTIONAL BRAIN

1. Deal with hyperactive arousal

Conventional psychiatry has used drugs to alter how we feel for years and its widely accepted to date. But we fail to push our being beyond what we can feel, we have what it takes and more residing in the inside to help conquer every depression and trauma. We can school our arousal system in ways we never thought was possible, even our breathing and movement can be trained to suit what you desire. This is possible because about eighty percent of the Vagus nerve fiber is afferent.

Asides the conventional usage of drugs and oral therapy, the following is helpful, movement, action, mindfulness, and rhythms (yoga, rhythmic drumming, martial arts, aikido, kendo, judo, jujitsu, tae kwon do, and capoeira). These practices involve breathing, physical movement, and meditation.

2. Be consciously mindful or else you will lose your mind -

To heal properly from trauma involves self-awareness. It gives you control over your anger, fear, and even anxiety and how you react to it. This way you are open to instruction and correction, you now react based on what is worth your while and not due to a senseless past habitual sensation.

When we mindfully connect to our feelings, we become more tolerating, bear discomfort as you know it's only for a little while, and reacts to un-expectancy aright instead of habitually freezing. Unlock the sensations you hid away because of the hurt it brings your way and let yourself feel it. The aim is to check how your body organizes certain emotions and the best way to deal with them.

3. Relationship

Socialization positively affects a traumatized person. It is a strong support network that protects against being traumatized. Relationship and human contact are warm and comforting and can never be downplayed. The faces and voices of familiar people you can trust are soothing and can be helpful to a survivor as well. Traumatized people need to be coached on how to be more open and trusting, everyone needs an anchor one time or the other in life.

In choosing a therapist, if they don't possess the following qualities you might have to keep searching – lay traumatic memories to rest, calm down troubled patients, connect patients with their colleagues. As a survivor, you can reach out to inquire of your therapist the strength of his skills, where he studied it, and if he has used his knowledge on trauma to help himself in the past.

4. Collective Rhythms and Synchrony

Trauma is a result of broken down attuned physical synchrony. There is strong healing power in communal music and rhythms. Music gives life, it was significantly expressed in 1997, during the Truth and Reconciliation Commission in Johannesburg, South Africa. Bessel attended a group of female rape survivors and life came back to the meeting because of rhythm. Other effective techniques of rhythm, movement, and touch were evident in Ying Mee who was mute but started talking after several failed attempts through the help of *sensory integration,* another is *Parent-child interaction therapy (PCIT).*

5. Be Touched

Medications such as reuptake blockers have been used over time to help people manage the happenings in their sensory world. But, touch is a far better option we rarely adopt. Touch is a natural therapy to help when in grief; being hugged, touched, and rocked insights a feeling of safety, protection, and control over your entire being.

6. Being in control

It is natural for the human body to secret stress hormones in response to responses to extreme experiences. Defenselessness and immobilization debar people from employing their stress hormones to protect themselves and because the action necessary for the pumped out hormone is yet to be utilized, the stress hormone keeps pumping. The result of that singular action results in incorrect freeze and fight/flight reactions. To gain back control over the body requires techniques such as cognitive-behavioral therapy (CBT), somatic experiencing, and sensorimotor psychotherapy.

DRUGS THAT ACCESS TRAUMA

The place of drugs cannot be ruled out. In 1985, MDMA (ecstasy) was adopted as a control substance as well as Effexor, Prozac, Paxil, Zoloft, and other psychotropic mediators (serotonin reuptake inhibitors (SSRIs))

MDMA reacts to some specific hormones like vasopressin, prolactin, oxytocin, and cortisol. It improves the awareness of self in various areas such as increased connectedness, compassionate energy, confidence, curiosity, creativity, and clarity. It reduces freezing feeling, defenselessness, and fear.

accompanied by curiosity, clarity, confidence, creativity, and connectedness. Research has it that patients who have been exposed to other forms of therapy and was futile tried MDMA in combination with psychotherapy and after two months, 83 percent of them were completely cured.

It's all about relationship and integration in turning a horrific event that takes the best of you into a memory of that occurred in the past. People aim to gain control of their entire being by using substances that block the pain and calms them down for a while but it always comes back. Substances like propranolol/clonidine (blocks the autonomic nervous system), cocaine, alcoholic drinks, tranquilizers like Klonopin, Valium and Xanax, cannabis, marijuana, and ganja. The desperation to be in control and calm drives people into this practice. When it wears out they are forced to take more and more and then get addicted which is a worse place to be in. Also in this place is antipsychotics, sedative-hypnotics, antidepressant, and other controlled substances.

Drugs cannot cure trauma nor does it train on long-term self-regulation. Recovery from trauma is not just a theory, it is achievable. Embrace your body, feel the feelings stirring inside of you, know why you feel that way, and gain back physical control of your life. Know that your memories don't control your reality, its only part of a progressing story.

- **Lessons**
    1. Neuroscience study expresses that the sure way we can alter the way we sense is to be aware of what we feel inside and learn to embrace it.
    2. It takes awareness of your traumatic episode to be in total control of your emotions.
- **Issues surrounding the subject matter**
    1. Are you comfortable with your therapist, his manner of treatment, and how effective is it and why?

_____

_____

_____

_____

_____

2. What changes have you noticed over time since you started your therapy session and do you feel you're being open to the therapist is helping or causing more havoc and why?

_____

_____

_____

_____

_____

3. Is control drugs bad over time and why?

_____

_____

_____

_____

- **Goals**
  1. How can one reach deep into their innate skills and discover the ways to live without control based drugs?

  _____

  _____

  _____

  _____

  2. In what ways can you embrace your emotional brain and how do you intend to work this out?

  _____

  _____

_____

_____

_____

3. How do you intend to take back ownership of your
   body, mind, and soul?

_____

_____

_____

_____

_____

- **Action steps**
  1. Mental health professionals, army sergeants, teachers,
  foster parents, are to be trained in emotional-regulation
  techniques.
- **Checklist**
  1. Drugs can never cure trauma.

CHAPTER 14
LANGUAGE: MIRACLE AND TYRANNY

In early 2002, Dr. Spencer Eth surveyed the traumatized survivors of the Twin Towers attack. They consisted of 225 people and he aimed to find out how the survivors were helped. The survivors attributed it to acupuncture, massage, yoga, and EMDR, and rescue workers credited it to massages.

Therapists believe so much in talking to cure trauma especially when the patient is open enough to divulge. But not all traumatized open up, it is harder than it sounds. It is quite difficult to express what your pain is in words but the pathway to resolving trauma begins with words and bit by bit the entire event comes to light. Keeping mute about your trauma is very lethal and can lead to death. Silence strengthens the isolating component of trauma. Speaking about your pain is relieving and a strong sign that you are ready to heal. Being able to find words to describe your Self in a language is agonizing, but when you can you are on the right track to self-discovery.

KNOWING YOURSELF OR TELLING YOUR STORY? OUR DUAL AWARENESS SYSTEM

Speaking about something that doesn't affect you personally can be so easy a topic for discussion but when it comes to relating your feelings in words, you discover how hard it can be. When we open up on our horrific past, it breaks your rigidity and opens us up to fresh opinions that are needed for survival.

Neuroscience reveals that humans possess two different forms of self-awareness located in two different parts of the brain: Autobiographical self (rooted in language, it keeps track of Self across time, builds connection amidst events, and arranges them in a clear story) and the other self-awareness is called moment-to-moment (rooted in physical sensation, one that registers Self in the present moment). The emotional brain can only be changed by the system dedicated to self-awareness which lays in the medial prefrontal cortex.

THE BODY IS THE BRIDGE

The stories of trauma reduce the separation trauma brings, it gives an excuse for the suffering experienced by the patients and why they do. With these stories, doctors can take note of possible diagnoses to address the root problem such as anger, insomnia, numbing, and nightmares. Stories give your blame a direction and a very good reason why a certain factor is been held accountable.

Other ways to effectively reach deep into your inner self is through writing, art, dance, and music. Writing to yourself blocks out the opinion others have of you. It doesn't matter what they say about you, write your truth down and read it to yourself and it will become what you desire. These techniques have helped many torture survivors, abused children, incest victims, soldiers suffering from PTSD, refugees, and more.

THE LIMITS OF LANGUAGE

Trauma devastates its listener as well as the speaker. It's not all the time that opening up about your trauma is embraced with open arms. Sometimes, divulging it alone can bring about rejection and hate. That's why it is often safe to speak in the presence of like minds – well trained professional therapist, like-minded group, etc. Working on traumatic memories is a good start at treating trauma. Patients with PTSD suffer first from a high level of deconcentrating and inability to learn new things.

A huge blunder of language is the thinking that our reasoning can be modified if it makes no sense. It's like trying to reframe negative conditions or turn the tables of the blame to suit the one who committed the atrocity. It cannot work. It is simply not done.

- **Lessons**
    1. Speaking about your pain is relieving and a strong sign that you are ready to heal.
    2. Being able to find words to describe your Self in a language is agonizing, but when you can you are on the right track to self-discovery.
    3. Trauma devastates its listener as well as the speaker.
- **Issues surrounding the subject matter**
    1. Why is it that it's not all the time that opening up about your trauma is embraced with open arms?

_____

_____

_____

_____

_____

- **Goals**
    1. How do trauma stories reduce the sequestration of trauma and provide a reason for why people suffer the way they do?

_____

_____

_____

_____

_____

2. In what ways do you think you will begin to be more open about your pain to resolve your trauma?

_____

_____

_____

_____

_____

- **Action steps**
   1. Apply this technique in solving the trauma of many survivors.
- **Checklist**
   1. Keeping mute about your trauma is very lethal and can lead to death.

CHAPTER 15

LETTING GO OF THE PAST: EMDR

Eye movement desensitization and reprocessing (EMDR) is a painful procedure that recreates the trauma of the past so that the patient can intentionally experience his feelings and relearn ways of controlling it.

EMDR was originated by psychologist Francine Shapiro after discovering that rapid eye movement incited a vivid relief from her misery. After several years of conducting tests and research, it is now an official standard procedure that can be tested and taught in controlled studies.

Bessel's EMDR training revealed some interesting things:

1. Its releases something in the mind that helps people to quickly reach slack related memories and images of the past.

2. It helps individuals observe their past in new ways without necessarily speaking about it and they get completely healed of the trauma.

3. It works whether the patient and therapist have a good rapport or not. This procedure is a great option for patients struggling very hard to divulge their pains and still want a solution.

4. Since patients don't have to speak about their hurt, they are fully focused on their internal experience with astonishing results from time to time.

5. The effectiveness of EMDR largely depends on the age the victim was abused leading to trauma. It plays a huge role in how susceptible the patient will receive the treatment.

6. EMDR numbs individuals of their traumatic contents thereby incorporating their traumatic material and links EMDR as a form of exposure therapy.

7. EMDR is seemingly related to the stage of sleep where dreaming takes place called – rapid eye movement (REM). Since this observation registered, it became a known fact that the more time derived from REM sleep eases depression and the reduced amount of REM sleep encourages depression.

8. EMDR doesn't waste time going back to visit the original trauma but concentrates on stimulating the divulging of the associative process.

- **Lessons**
  1. Eye movement desensitization and reprocessing (EMDR) is a painful procedure that recreates the trauma of the past so that the patient can intentionally experience his feelings and relearn ways of controlling it.

- **Issues surrounding the subject matter**
  1. Can EMDR make it harmless for individuals to gain entrance into the trajectories of trauma and then turn them into memories of experiences that occurred in the past?

———————————————————————

———————————————————————

———————————————————————

———————————————————————

_____

_____

2. What are your reservations as regards EMDR, as many seem to be doubtful of its excessively good to be true and too simple to be so powerful attributes?

_____

_____

_____

_____

_____

_____

- **Goals**
  1. How can people reach back into their traumatic past short of being re-traumatized all over again?

  _____

  _____

  _____

  _____

  _____

- **Action steps**
  1. Approach EMDR with an open heart erasing all doubts.
- **Checklist**
  1. Memories develop and modifies after every telling of your experience and are prone to reinterpretation and integration.

CHAPTER 16
LEARNING TO INHABIT YOUR BODY: YOGA

THE LEGACY OF INESCAPABLE SHOCK

Faulty alarm systems reveal itself in many ways and this malfunction in the smoke detector makes your perception unreliable and inaccurate. Trauma experience puts a person in two separate states of consciousness. The victim still lives in shock and blame themselves for their state and suffering even when their rational mind tells them otherwise. This conflict is a result of the emotional brain as wired by the limbic system.

THE NUMBING WITHIN

With the increase in muscle tension or sensing of disintegration in the trauma center part of the body; be it the vagina for sexual abuse survivors, the back, neck, limb for accident victims, or any other body part as the case may be is all as a result of stored memory of helplessness. A traumatized person gains their life back when they can withstand and silence unwanted sensory experiences. Constant muscle tension results in migraines, spasms, headaches, back pains, and other chronic pain. Medications for soothing these level of pain doesn't solve the problem or aims to find the root cause, all it can offer is temporary happiness after which the body begins to suffer all over again.

FINDING OUR WAY TO YOGA: BOTTOM-UP REGULATION

The heart rate variability (HRV) is a good tool to help in measuring the functionality and workings of the autonomic nervous system which is the brain's primary survival system whose two branches are responsible for triggering arousal all over the body. A balanced autonomic nervous system is a state where the sympathetic nervous system (SNS) and the parasympathetic nervous system (PNS) are functioning optimally. With this balance in mind, individuals will assume control over their reaction to minute disappointment and be calm when insulted or trampled on. Research has it that HRV can be increased in the following way;

a. Marathon running
b. Yoga
c. Martial art
d. Qigong

Yoga helps individuals discover internal balance and keeps them in their topmost shape of health. Science also made it known that altering one's breathing can positively improve their medical state. Illnesses like increased hormonal secretion, high blood pressure, lower back pain, and even asthma. Yoga improves HRV in the area of breathing synchronically to give the heart a rhythm that is cardiac coherent.

Yoga's effect on psychological functioning improves arousal tremendously in PTSD patients and significantly improves the survivor's relationship to their physical body. Today, yoga programs have been infused in trauma therapy such as meditations, breath practices (pranayama), and postures/stretches. This is all in a bid to encourage mindfulness so as patients take different poses they are intentionally taking note of what is happening in their body during the stance.

Yoga has different poses and some patients report how it makes them vulnerable and they tend to remember their painful past; but the sooner they can self-regulate these events so that the memory of it doesn't hurt them anymore; they will still be in bondage.

LEARNING TO COMMUNICATE

The only way we can successfully communicate is when we feel safe in our bodies and translate the memories that formerly overwhelmed us into language.

- **Lessons**
  1. Yoga can alter HRV
  2. The practice of yoga made it easy for people to believe in themselves.
  3. The increase in muscle tension or sensing of disintegration in the trauma center part of the body; be it the vagina for sexual abuse survivors, the back, neck, limb for accident victims, or any other body part as the case may be is all as a result of stored memory of helplessness.
- **Issues surrounding the subject matter**
  1. How can one patient recover from trauma and still be in a state of complete relaxation and safety?

  _____

  _____

  _____

  _____

  _____

- **Goals**
  1. How can people improve their HRV?

  _____

  _____

  _____

_____

_____

2. How can you learn to experience your feelings without being transfixed by them?

_____

_____

_____

_____

_____

3. Does yoga make you tolerant to touch, how and why?

_____

_____

_____

_____

_____

- **Action steps**
    1. The only way we can successfully communicate is when we feel safe in our bodies and translate the memories that formerly overwhelmed us into language.
- **Checklist**
    1. Yoga practice increases your self-awareness.

CHAPTER 17

PUTTING THE PIECES TOGETHER: SELF-LEADERSHIP

Some traumatized persons display dissociative identity disorder (DID) where an individual processes dual identities. Everyone has conflicting impulses but that of a traumatized person is extreme just for survival purposes. Embracing/exploring both parts is an intrinsic component of healing.

DESPERATE TIMES REQUIRE DESPERATE MEASURES

Situations just like a trauma that makes us aim to protect ourselves at all times and an increased desire to survive at all costs just like humiliation trigger feelings of anger, revenge, and wanting to become more successful and powerful so that you will not be a subject of ridicule next time. These sorts of situations can bring about behaviors to make yourself look tough and invincible such as; compulsion, self-destructive behavior, obsession, and also panic attacks which all began all in a bid to protect Self. Patients resort to medications to help them manage their crisis and they use these medications for what seems like forever because the drug is not a curative measure.

For traumatic memories that intrude the mind at any given time and changes the hormonal balance to the system to attack itself, until the incorporates all its part and feel safe in itself, it will never stop fighting nor stop living in trauma.

The human mind is a medley of different personalities and potentialities that makes it complex though still functions as one body. On the other hand, the traumatic mind disintegrates and wars with one another making the body constantly remind in an aggressive fight/flight mode. We have to take good care of our health, lingering problems get in the way of our reaching our internal properties. The therapists are to join forces with the survivor instead of schooling or trying to fix stuff in the holes the trauma created. Mindfully embrace your vulnerabilities as all your parts work in sync to accomplish one major goal and that is to protect it from harm. This is where mindful self-leadership comes to play which is a huge stepping stone and bedrock to be healed of your trauma.

The concept of mindfulness by Schwartz as it concerns dynamic leadership is that Self doesn't need cultivating or developing as there is as a part in every human and even trauma victim that can never be destroyed that is calm, confident, curious, and protected from destruction to guarantee survival. Secondly, the mindful Self increases control over the amygdala by reforming the inner system and disseminate the information to the other parts that there is no cause for alarm and that the system can be trusted.

GETTING TO KNOW THE INTERNAL LANDSCAPE

Therapist help patents achieve the following;

- Isolate the mystifying balance into unconnected entities.
- Inspire patients to inquire of each defensive part to be sure of what they are protecting and make room for mindful self-observation.
- They help patients recognize the portion responsible for their present predicament.

There are firefighters, exiles, and managers. The firefighter guards and protects the system while the manager is calm and collected and cooperative in therapy.

THE POWER OF SELF-COMPASSION: IFS IN THE TREATMENT OF RHEUMATOID ARTHRITIS

Nancy Shadick, a rheumatologist at Boston's Brigham and Richard Schwartz discovered IFS (Internal Family System) to help in treating rheumatoid arthritis (RA) patients. The result of their nine-months research period revealed that IFS resulted in significant improvements in self-compassion, self-efficacy, joint pain, depression, and overall physical and mental pain of the patient. This is so because research has it that cognitive behavior psychoanalysis and mindfulness-based practices positively impact depression, pain, physical disability, and joint inflammation.

This study tremendously shows that RA can be helped by psychological interventions.

- **Lessons**
    1. Rheumatoid arthritis can be helped by psychological interventions.
    2. Patients are to mindfully embrace their vulnerabilities as all the body parts work in sync to accomplish one major goal and that is to protect it from harm.
- **Issues surrounding the subject matter**
    1. Do you deal with your dissociative identity disorder (DID) or you embrace it?

_____

_____

_____

_____

_____

- **Goals**

1. Does increased mental security and wellbeing result in an enhanced-functioning immune system and why?

_____

_____

_____

_____

_____

- **Action steps**

  1. The therapists are to join forces with the survivor instead of schooling or trying to fix stuff in the holes the trauma created.

- **Checklist**

  1. Embrace and explore both dual personalities because it is an intrinsic component of healing.

CHAPTER 18

FILLING IN THE HOLES: CREATING STRUCTURES

Deciphering the memories of trauma is one thing and a different ball game to face the internal emptiness caused by trauma, the neglect, not being wanted, not wanted to be seen or spoken nor to speak the truth. It is difficult to learn a feeling you have never experienced since childhood and now introduced at an advanced age. This is so because there is no memory of what is newly introduced to latch on and reactivate what already existed although numb due to some factors.

Patients who have been abused can move on with their lives if only they can rebuild their inherent maps. This involves being intuitively conversant with the feelings that are absent when they were quite younger.

Ex-dancer with the Martha Graham Dance Company – Albert Pesso discovered a way to alter the amygdala (people's relationship) to their fundamental self even though there was no scientific backing then, he was still unwavering. He used micro-tracking to keep track of everybody's language, tone, posture, eye gaze, and facial expression of his participant as he sat beside. Once in a while, Albert makes a witness statement during the PBSP psychomotor therapy session that makes his subject calmer, more divulging and relaxed to go deeper into the nitty-gritty of her horrific ordeal, as time passes he requests if the subjects need succor in form of a person just to "register" a contact person and when they affirm they got.

As the subject told her story, significant people in the patient's life were acted right in front of her in montages, this helped her inner world take the three-dimensional (realistic) cosmos. The recreating of their past made it look real and established a kind of connection that would ignite the right emotion responsible for their pain and be tackled accordingly.

RESTRUCTURING INNER MAPS

Acting out the images going on in your mind via spatial right in front of you gives you a clearer picture of what resides in your mind and better ways to react to others and yourself about your past. The presentation of your life story can be manipulated like a chess piece on the board.

With your life history laid bare in front of you, you have the opportunity to decide how you react and reform the damages your past caused. This way you make new memories in the present and the past remains in history. This new memory doesn't erase the past, but it gives you a healthy option to choose from. The psychomotor therapy helps to provide a cure for painful memories by making virtual memories that live alongside past painful realities and provide physical experiences of all you crave as remedies to hurtful memories.

- **Lessons**
  1. Patients who have been abused can move on with their lives if only they can rebuild their inherent maps. This involves being intuitively conversant with the feelings that are absent when they were quite younger.
- **Issues surrounding the subject matter**
  1. For patients that are new to certain feelings been taught, how can they learn to love, trust and care and reciprocate when they have never experienced it before?

_____

_____

_____

_____

_____

- **Goals**
  1. How can patients who have been abused move on with their lives by rebuilding their inherent maps?

  _____

  _____

  _____

  _____

  _____

  2. How can using psychomotor therapy help to a cure for painful memories by making virtual memories?

  _____

  _____

  _____

  _____

  _____

- **Action steps**
  1. Adopt the use of PBSP psychomotor therapy to build new memories you can refer to when the past creeps in.
- **Checklist**
  1. The demonstration of your life story can be manipulated like a chess piece on the board.

CHAPTER 19

REWIRING THE BRAIN: NEUROFEEDBACK

During Bessel's freelance at the Boston State Hospital as a research assistant for Ernest Hartmann's sleep laboratory in his first year of medical school, his duty was to organize and monitor the study members in other to examine their EEG (electroencephalogram) OR brain wave. Electrodes and wires were strapped to their scalp and eyes for monitoring rapid eye movements (REM) and to check the brain activity when the body is asleep. It was significantly clear that the neurons in the brain still communicated and this was conveyed to the polygraph set aside for the study. When the polygraph records a REM sleep cycle by the subjects, they are then woken up and asked what they dreamt of and it is recorded and a questionnaire is drafted from the findings to ascertain sleep quality.

MAPPING THE ELECTRICAL CIRCUITS OF THE BRAIN

In the past, it was believed that brain activity relied on both electrical and chemical signals. Later Hans Berger a German Psychiatrist recorded the first brain's electrical activity in 1924 which was met with a lot of cynicism and scorn by the medical institution. Not long after, electroencephalography became an essential tool to make a diagnosis of seizure activity in individuals with epilepsy. Berger found out that different mental activities are due to various brain-wave patterns with the hope that one-day science would be able to associate different psychiatric problems with specific electroencephalogram irregularities.

In 2000 a breakthrough in the disparity in fact processing amongst distressed subjects and a collection of "normal" Australians was conducted using "the oddball paradigm" which is a standardized test. The test required patients to detect items not suitable in a chain of otherwise connected images. The result was clear as the brains of the individuals in the normal group worked collectively to make a rational pattern of focus, filtering, and analysis. On the other hand, the brains of the traumatized people were inaccurately coordinated and didn't make a comprehensible pattern. This simply means that their brain couldn't make a brainwave pattern to enable them to be attentive and separate relevant and irrelevant information.

This lack of attention and focus common with patients of PTSD is due to the malfunction of the brain-wave pattern. In 2007 Sebern Fisher an ex-clinical director of a residential treatment center for traumatized youths revealed how neurofeedback has helped her achieve a lot of breakthroughs for the adolescents.

SEEING THE SYMPHONY OF THE BRAIN

Sebern conducts her neurofeedback remedy using 2 desktop computers along with a small amplifier and then attaches an electrode to each side of the skull and one on the right ear. The computer will display brain waves portraying the electrical symphony of my brain. This function mirrors the activities going on in the brain. Neurofeedback allows for the brain to create more beneficial frequencies and new patterns diminish others just to enhance the brain's natural intricacy and its preference to self-regulation. Neurofeedback can trail the electrical system in certain parts of the brain.

Using neurofeedback to cure trauma requires going through the circuitry of the brain and correct and stabilize the organs that promote the sustained level of fear, anger, and shame. When the brain pattern goes back to the status quo it originally was in, everything goes back to normal and there will not be a need to extremities in the hormonal display or physical actions.

GETTING STARTED IN NEUROFEEDBACK AND ITS BENEFITS

Different neurofeedback systems should be adopted after a series of test to know which is suitable to a patient such as;

1. Hem encephalography (HEG)
2. SMR (traditional)
3. QEEG (quantitative electroencephalography)
4. Alpha/Theta (A/T)
5. Coherence training
6. Neuro-Gen HPN
7. Beta Reset
8. Interactive Metronome

BENEFITS OF NEUROFEEDBACK;

- It helps the brain focus, concentration, and attention
- increase creativity
- improve athletic control
- enhances inner awareness
- improves musical performance
- improves learning abilities and comprehension
- helps in fighting off PTSD symptoms and addictions such as drug abuse, alcohol abuse, etc.
- helpful for hyperarousal and confusion challenges.
- Helps in easing tension
- Eases anxiety and panic attack

- Teats autism
- Better control for seizure
- helps the cerebral function in recuperating after a distressing brain injury
  - **Lessons**
    1. Neurofeedback can trail the electrical system in certain parts of the brain thereby giving it a fighting chance to correct the faults up there.
    2. Today neurofeedback is used in treating patients with PTSD.
  - **Issues surrounding the subject matter**
    1. How do you think electrical brain activity contributes to psychiatric problems?

    _____

    _____

    _____

    _____

    _____

    2. What are the ways to repair dysfunctional brain-wave patterns?

    _____

    _____

    _____

    _____

    _____

  - **Goals**
    1. In what ways can neurofeedback aid the elimination of trauma in a traumatized person?

_____

_____

_____

_____

_____

- **Action steps**

    1. Make sure your therapist has done all the findings necessary before recommending neurofeedback for you.

- **Checklist**

    1. Using neurofeedback to cure trauma requires going through the circuitry of the brain.

CHAPTER 20
FINDING YOUR VOICE: COMMUNAL RHYTHMS AND THEATER

Our entire being, association, the level of our command, and what we command, how we walk, sit, eat, and sleep is largely dependent on our relationship with our physical bodies and rhythms. Finding our voice means discovering our true essence and that can only be done when we are inside our bodies.

To find your voice; every iota of disassociation will be put to an end, it all starts by acting what you want your life to look like even though it may not seem like it at the onset, it will make sense later.

TREATING TRAUMA THROUGH THEATER

Theater programs have a way of helping to alleviate the effect of trauma on traumatized people. There are various therapeutic drama programs, the idea is a breakout from being controlled by fear, anger, and numbness. The infusion of theatrical dexterity is to make you face the things you are scared of the most; your family conflicts, internal conflicts, social conflicts, interpersonal conflicts which are all attributes in drama.

In theater there is no hiding your fears, anger, and helplessness; the verity of your deep truth will always come out. It is not easy to open up about your horrific past but forcing your way through the hurt to find out your truth and examine what is going on inside of you to find your voice and be comfortable in your own body.

This program isn't for experts, they are meant for angry, scared, and crumbling individuals who are evidently out of sync with their bodies and need harmony back in their lives. Examples of exercises conducted for trauma drama programs;

- Dialogue with the back (goal is to lead the way amongst group members which will elicit various emotions)
- Playing in pairs (inspires creativity, teamwork, and impulsiveness)
- What's in a Name? (develops their imaginative abilities and creativity)
- Mirroring reverberation (participant are guided on their internal conflict from a new viewpoint, improve their listening skill, and learn to work harmoniously with others)
- Reunion (participants improvise and act in the future)

- **Lessons**
  1. Finding our voice means discovering our true essence and that can only be done when we are inside our bodies.
- **Issues surrounding the subject matter**
  1. Is it a must for patients to go through theatrical trauma programs to be completely cured of their trauma?

_____
_____
_____
_____
_____

- **Goals**
  1. How can you ensure that drama therapy programs are infused in the school curriculum, prisons, and other agencies?

  _____
  _____
  _____
  _____
  _____
  _____
  _____
  _____
  _____
  _____

- **Action steps**

  1. Your driving force is the fact that you want to feel better and end the torture.

- **Checklist**

  1. In theater there is no hiding your fears, anger, and helplessness; the verity of your deep truth will always come out.

CONCLUSION
CHOICES TO BE MADE

Daily, many people are losing their minds, falling into trauma, and losing touch of their body and life in general. Early abuse wrecks the life, social operation, and health of a promising child that if not addressed on time can be very difficult to redress in the future.

With the reduction in sexual abuse, domestic violence, troubled homes, violence, war, crime, and trauma inciting experiences, the world will be a better place and we will experience less pain. With the help of neuroscience, we can now tell how trauma alters the development of the brain and its inability to stay focused. Techniques have also revealed the parts of the brain that is affected by trauma leading to PTSD and the measures to adopt to get a solution.

Asides from popular cases of trauma, there are others not often projected that live with us daily and haunt us such as politics. This terminology largely determines how far one goes in life, once the government has its people at heart; things will go on in their favor. Its decisions affect our housing, educational opportunities, income, employment, health opportunities, and even family structure. Basic amenities that are every human's right can make life meaningless and unpleasant. Other drawbacks are unemployment, social isolation, poverty, inferior school, crime, and poor housing can translate quickly into trauma if not addressed sooner.

As humans, we are wired to connect and socialize. The long-term nonexistence of that shows something wrong in the entire body system. With time the body parts begin to collapse one after the other due to the inactivity and dwelling in the past for longer than necessary. Survivors are to learn to control their behavior and not shy away from new and possible solutions. Medications for trauma is for temporary relief, you need to be back in sync with your entire being by embracing what you feel internal and assume control over yourself.

Therapists and teachers should on the other hand take it easy with these children who display trauma like tantrums. Calm the child down and inquire why he/she is upset and proffer a possible solution. It is wrong to swing into action first by reprimanding and even beating the child, which can worsen the child's state. Self-regulation, emotional intelligence, and passionate communal effort should be inculcated in training kids and adult as well.

Lightning Source UK Ltd.
Milton Keynes UK
UKHW021847131220
374938UK00003B/366